Majdi Ben Romdhane
Rafik Elafram
Majdi Sghaier

HUMERAL SHAFT FRACTURES: THERAPEUTIC ALTERNATIVES

HUMERAL SHAFT FRACTURES: THERAPEUTIC ALTERNATIVES

Majdi Ben Romdhane
Rafik Elafram
Majdi Sghaier

HUMERAL SHAFT FRACTURES: THERAPEUTIC ALTERNATIVES

ScienciaScripts

have long after-effects, fraught with complications, without leading to definitive consolidation, necessitating the use of different therapeutic techniques, with repeated failures that are sometimes accepted even as irrecoverable. Numerous therapeutic methods have been proposed, ranging from orthopaedic immobilisation techniques to surgery. These include screw-plate osteosynthesis, endomedullary osteosynthesis (fasciculated pinning or nailing), and external fixation.In reality, the effectiveness of each of these methods is only complete in the long term if their execution technique has been respected from the outset. For humeral shaft fractures, fasciculated pinning is the technique most prone to post-operative complications, such as delayed consolidation, callus, pseudarthrosis, radial paralysis and stiffness of the shoulder and elbow. While the screw plate represents the gold standard for surgical treatment, since in addition to the absence of post-operative immobilisation and early resumption of work, this technique offers the best functional results with a low risk of damage to the radial nerve. Centromedullary nailing is an interesting alternative with intermediate post-operative results.

For type B or C fractures according to the AO [5], we opt for

For type A fractures, the indications are divided between fasciculated pinning and centromedullary nailing.

In order to gain a better understanding of the problems posed by these diaphyseal fractures, this study was based on a literature review of the various surgical techniques. The most commonly used classification is that of the AO[5].

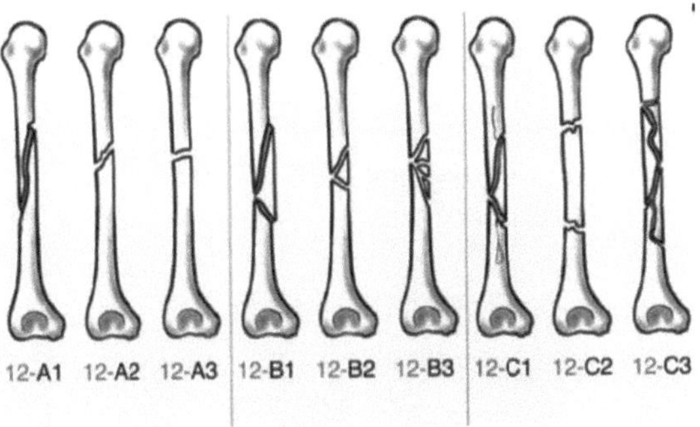

AO/OTA classification of diaphyseal humeral fractures.

Figure 1: AO classification for diaphyseal fractures of the the humerus

The 3 most commonly used techniques are as follows:

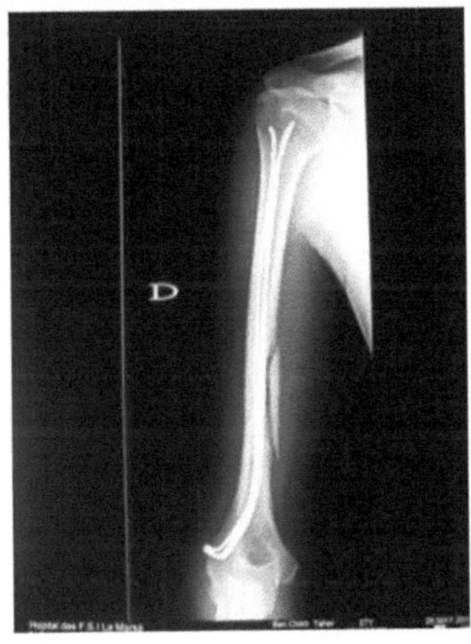

1. Fasciculated packaging
2. Figure 2: Reduction without inter-fragment gap

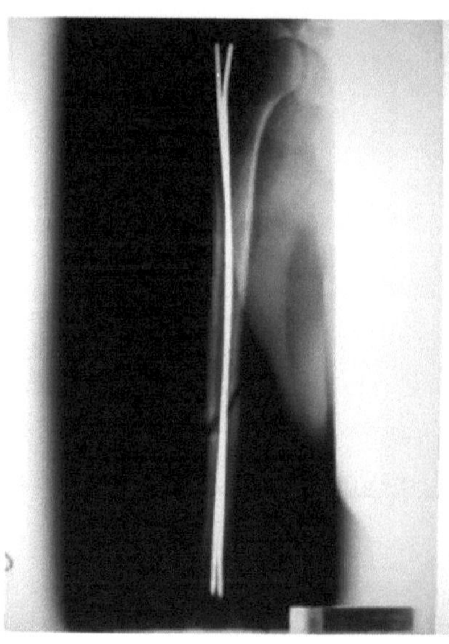

Figure 3: Fasciculated pin reduction with inter-fragmentary gap

The patient is positioned supine, arms resting on a radiolucent table, with the amplifier placed at the patient's head.The approach is made via a longitudinal incision strictly centred on the relief of the lateral epicondyle, with the epicondylar muscles removed over a distance of a few millimetres; the medullary cavity is entered by directing the square tip obliquely at 45° upwards and slightly posteriorly through an entry point just above the apophysis; the orifice is then enlarged at the expense of the posterolateral edge of the humeral palette in this lateral epicondylar approach, the radial nerve is far from the approach.The essential condition for this operation is that the fracture must be reducible in a closed setting. Once this has been achieved and maintained either by the operating aid and the entry window When the procedure is carried out, the pins are inserted from distal to proximal. An image intensifier is used to check the passage of the fracture site and the cephalic divergence of the wires. Large diameter Kirschner wires are used and endomedullary cortical filling: a compromise must be found between the possibilities of future extraction and the absence of conflict with the soft tissues. The cortical window is cut at the expense of the posterior surface of the external pillar of the humeral pallet, i.e. 2 to 3 cm above the relief of the lateral epicondyle.

3. Plate osteosynthesis

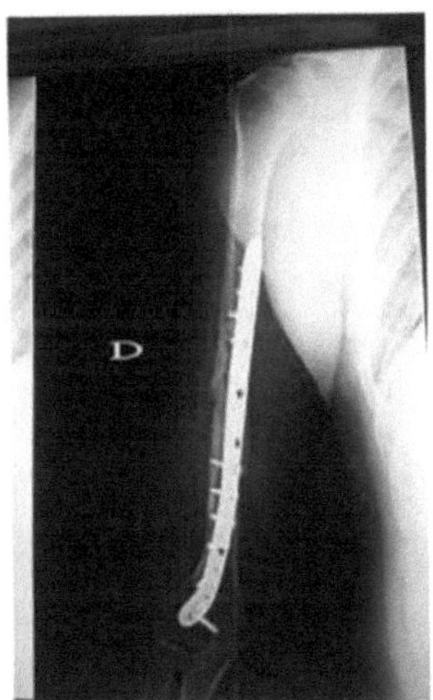

Figure 4: Screw plate reduction

a. Installing the patient :
The patient is positioned supine, with the arm resting on a hand-held table.

b. Surgical approach :
The skin incision forms a parenthesis, curving forwards towards the distal deltopectoral groove and the upper part of the lateral bicipital groove. The external intermuscular partition is the first element to be identified: the radial nerve pierces it from front to back before slipping between the biceps and the long suppinator. It is the first nerve to be found and placed on the lac. It is not always easy to find: do not hesitate

to palpate the muscle fibres directly to feel it "roll", or look for it more distally in the bicipital groove. No traction should be exerted on it; this is a constant concern for the surgeon and his assistant.

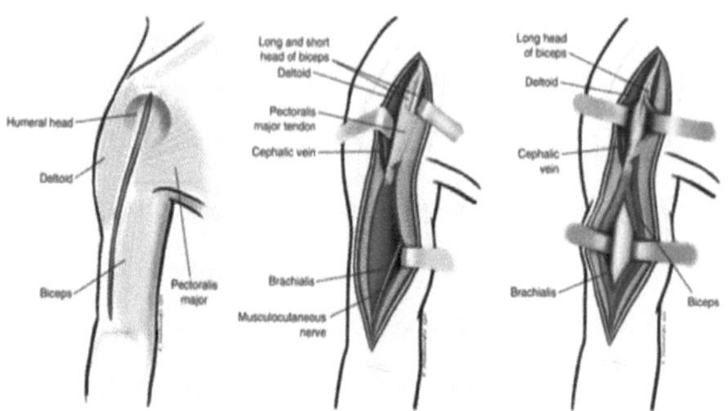

Figure 5: antero-external approach to the upper arm

The muscles of the anterior compartment are roughened, exposing the anterolateral surface of the diaphysis on which the plate is placed. A forceps is used for reduction; in the case of oblique, spiral or "butterfly wing" lines In the case of an oblique, spiral or "butterfly wing" line, one or more 4.5 or 3.5 mm compression screws are used, with the cortical bone under the screw head being drilled to the same diameter. The plate is then selected, comprising at least three cortices on either side of the focal point, under compression using the staggered screw hole system. The incision is external longitudinal; the radial nerve, after crossing the intermuscular septum, is sought distally between the anterior brachial and brachioradialis.

4. Centromedullary nailing

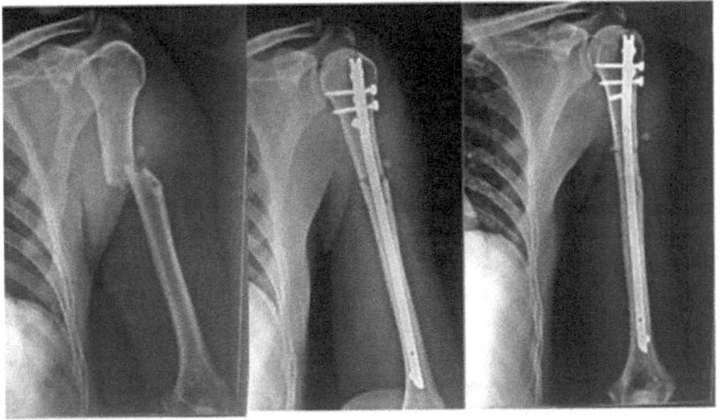

Figure 6: Centromedullary nailing

a- Installing the patient :

For proximo-distal nailing, the upper limb should protrude above the table to be manipulated and to allow the amplifier to be controlled. Some people recommend a semi-seated position [6].

b- First is the point of introduction:

The approach to the spinal cord is via an anterolateral incision of 3 to 4 cm at the acromial margin. There is some disagreement as to where the nail should be inserted.Seidel[7] recommends a radial incision in the cuff tendon insertion zone and lateral bone penetration, at the major cartilage-tubercle junction. Kempf [8] positions the incision extra-articularly, i.e. more laterally; at the top of the trochiter. Conversely, Riemer [9] recommends a more medial radial incision of the cuff and a bony approach in the same axis as the medullary cavity, the projection of which ends in the cephalic epiphyseal cartilage medial to the trochle.

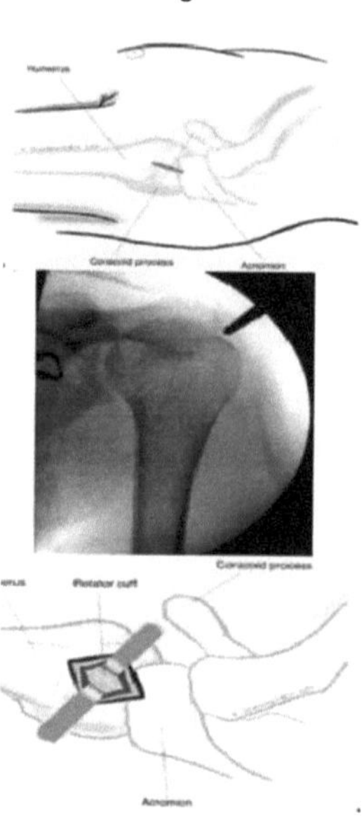

Figure 7: Approach and preparation of nail entry EPIDEMIOLOGICAL STUDY

I. EPIDEMIOLOGY

I.1. Age :

In series published in the literature [10-13] , the mean age of was 36.27
years.

Table 1: Average age of patients.

Author	Average age
N. Nachef [10]	39,94
M. Barsaoui [11]	38
O. Mohamed [12]	29
O. Margad [13]	35

I.2. Gender :

In the literature [13-15] , the sex ratio was 4.66

Table 2: Sex ratio of humeral shaft fractures.

Author	Sex ratio
D. Ring [23]	3
O. Margad [22]	6
RL. Sahu [24]	5

I.3. Achieved :

The left side was most frequently affected in the literature [12, 13, 16]; in the series by B. Cherif [20], the right side was most frequently affected,

Table 3: The affected side in humeral shaft fractures.

Author	Side reached
C.B Diémé [16]	left
O. Margad [13]	left
O. Mohamed [12]	left

I.4. Circumstances of occurrence :

In the literature, road traffic accidents were the most frequent cause in young subjects [10, 12, 13]. In elderly subjects, falls were the most frequent cause [10, 17].

Table 4: Circumstances of onset of diaphyseal fractures.

Author	Circumstances of occurrence
H. Bèzes [18]	AS
T. Flinkkilâ [17]	Drop
N. Nachef [10]	AVP/Chute
O. Mohamed [12]	AVP
O. Margad [13]	AVP

II. PREOPERATIVE RESULTS

II.1. Study of the fracture :

II.1.1. Head office:

In series published in the literature, the middle third of the humeral diaphysis was the preferred site in 57.31% of cases [10-14, 16, 18, 19].

Table 5: Location of humeral shaft fractures.

Author	Location
M. Barsaoui [11]	middle third
D. Ring [14]	middle third
H. Bèzes [18]	middle third
C.B Diémé [16]	middle third
O. Margad [13]	middle third
K. Singisetti [19]	middle third
O. Mohamed [12]	middle third
N. Nachef [10]	middle third-distal third junction

II.1.2. Type of line :

In the literature, the most frequent fractures were type A [10-14, 16, 19].

Table 6: Type of line according to the A0 classification of humeral shaft fractures.

Author	Type of line (AO)
K. Singisetti [19]	A/B
O. Margad [13]	A
N. Nachef [10]	A
O.Mohamed [12]	A
D. Ring [14]	A
M. Barsaoui [11]	A
C.B Diémé [16]	A

II.2. Local associated lesions :

II.2.1. Skin opening :

In the series by N. Nachef [10], 1/17 of the cases were complicated by an open type I Gustilo fracture. In the series by D. Ring [14], these were high-energy traumas. In the literature The rate of open fractures was 14.81% of cases [10-14], the most frequent of which were Gustilo type 1.

Table 7: Frequency of open humeral shaft fractures according to the Gustilo classification.

Author	Skin opening	Type I	Type II	Type III
D. Ring [14]	11/24	0	5	6
M. arsaoui 11]	13/70	7	4	2
O. ohamed [12]	2/54	1	0	0
O. Margad [13]	4/80	2	2	0
N. Nachef [10]	1/17	1	0	0

II.2.2. Initial radial paralysis :

In the literature, radial nerve injuries were found in 18.68% of cases [11-13, 16, 18-20]. The fractures were at the from third middle (60%) [10-14, 16, 18, 19] Thisanatomical peculiarity explains these results.

Table 8: Frequency of initial radial paralysis in humeral shaft fractures.

Author	Radial paralysis
O. Mohamed [12]	3/51
O. Margad [13]	6/80
C.B. Diémé [16]	5/58
M. Barsaoui [11]	7/70
H. Bèzes [18]	26/236
K. Singisetti [19]	4/36
J. Robert [20]	9/14

II.3. Polytrauma :

In the literature, 24.65% of humeral shaft fractures were polytraumatic. [12-14, 16, 18, 20] For D. Ring [14], these were high-energy traumas and 8/24 polytraumas were found.

Table 9: Frequency of polytrauma in humeral shaft fractures.

Author	Polytrauma
C.B. Diémé [16]	9/600
H. Bèzes [18]	66/253
D. Ring [14]	8/24
J. Robert [20]	13/14
O. Mohamed [12]	5/51
O. Margad [13]	8/70

III. TREATMENT

III.1. Operating time :

In series published in the literature, the average operating time was 5 days [11-13].

Table 10: Average operating time for humeral shaft fractures.

Author	Average operating time (days)
O. Margad [13]	4
M. Barsaoui [11]	3,7
O. Mohamed [12]	3,4

III.2. General anaesthesia :

In the series by C.B. Diémé [16], 46/58 cases were operated on under general anaesthesia. In the literature,90.51% of patients were operated on under general anaesthetic [12, 13, 15, 16, 21].

Table 11: Frequency of humeral shaft fractures operated on under general anaesthetic.

Author	General anaesthesia
RL. Sahu [15]	78/78
B. D'ythurbide [21]	57/57
O. Margad [13]	68/70
O. Mohamed [12]	34/51
C.B Diémé [16]	46/58

III.3. Type of surgery :

III.3.1. Screw-on plate :

In the series by K. Singisetti [19], 16/26 patients underwent screw-plate surgery. In the literature, fractures operated on with a screw-plate were of type A [10, 18, 19, 22].

Table 12: Humeral shaft fractures operated on with screw plates.

Author	Number of cases	Type of fracture
H. Bèzes [18]	246/246	A1
N. Nachef [10]	17/17	A1
AB. Putti [22]	18/34	A3
K. Singisetti [19]	16/36	A3/B2

III.3.2. Centromedullary nailing :

In the literature, fractures treated by centromedullary nailing were type A [15, 19, 21-23].

Table 13: Humeral shaft fractures operated on by centromedullary nailing.

Author	Number of cases	Type of fracture
B. D'ythurbide [21]	57/57	A3
RL. Sahu [15]	78/78	A1
M.J.G Blyth [23]	50/50	A1
K. Singisetti [19]	20/36	A3/B2
AB. Putti [22]	16/34	A3

III.3.3. Percutaneous embrochage :

In the literature, fractures treated by percutaneous pinning accounted for 79.90% of cases [12, 13, 16].In the literature, fractures treated by percutaneous pinning were type A [12, 13, 16].

Table 14: Humeral shaft fractures operated on by percutaneous pinning.

Author	Number of cases	Type of fracture
O. Mohamed [12]	51/51	A3
C.B Diémé [16]	58/58	A3
O. Margad [13]	70/70	A3

IV. POSTOPERATIVE RESULTS

The results of the quality of the initial reduction in the literature are very similar [12, 13]

Table 15: Quality of initial reduction in the literature

Author	Good reduction	Wrong reduction	Nb of case
O. Mohamed [12]	51	0	51
O. Margad [13]	60	10	50

V.RESULTS AT LAST RETREAT

V.1. The latest setback :

In the literature, the mean follow-up was 23.17 months [10-12, 15].

Table 16: Average recoil of humeral shaft fractures.

Author	Average backlog (months)
O. Mohamed [12]	45
N. Nachef [10]	31
M. Barsaoui [11]	20
RL. Sahu [15]	9

V.2. Results by technique :

V.2.1. Screw-on plate :

V.2.1.1. Consolidation :

In the literature, the rate of consolidation in fractures operated on with a screw-plate was 85.38% [19, 24]; in the series by JR. Chapman [24] is 16 weeks.

Table 17: Consolidation of humeral shaft fractures treated with screw plates.

Author	Number of cases	consolidation (%)	Deadline of consolidation (weeks)
JR Chapman [24]	46/84	43/46	16
K. Singisetti [19]	16/36	12/16	16

V.2.1.2. Complications :

V.2.1.2.1. Sepsis :

In the series by AB. Putti [22], 1/34 of the fractures treated with screw plates were complicated by sepsis.

V.2.1.2.2. Radial paralysis :

In the series by K. Singisetti, there was 1 case of radial paralysis secondary to treatment with a screw-plate [19], involving a type A2 fracture in the lower third of the humeral shaft. Intraoperatively, the radial nerve was contused and treatment was with a Lecestre-type plate. Post-operative immobilisation was of the Mayo Clinic type for a period of 21 days.This radial nerve paralysis recovered after 6 months.

V.2.1.2.3. Pseudarthrosis :

In the literature, the incidence of pseudarthrosis after treatment with screw plates was 6.05% [10, 18, 19, 22, 25]. For H. Bèzes [18], pseudarthrosis on screw plates is often due to poor synthesis: absence of compression or interfragmentary gap on the side opposite the plate, a plate that is too thin, or a number of screws that is too small. insufficient, resulting in an unstable assembly.

V.2.1.2.4. Delayed consolidation :

In the literature, the incidence of delayed consolidation in cases treated with screw plates is 5.68% [10, 18, 19, 22, 25].

V.2.1.2.5. Cal vicious :

No vicious callus was found in fractures treated with screw plates in the literature [10, 18, 19, 22, 25].

Table 18: Complications in humeral shaft fractures treated with screw plates.

Author	No. of cases	Sepsis	Paralysis Radials	Pseudarthrosis	Delay in Consolidation	Cal Vicieux
H. Bèzes [18]	246/246	2/246	5/246	3/246	0	0
N.Nachef[10]	17/17		4/17	0	0	0
M.B Gottschalk [25]	2560/3430		201/2560	45/2560	0	0
AB. Putti [22]	18/34	1/18	0	0	0	0
K.Singisetti [19]	16/36		1/16	1/16	4/16	0

V.2.2. Centromedullary nailing :

V.2.2.1. Consolidation :

In the literature, the rate of consolidation in fractures operated on by centromedullary nailing was 84.59% [15, 19, 23], with an average time to consolidation of 22.93 weeks, with a minimum time to consolidation in the series by K. Singisetti [19] (16 weeks) and a maximum in the series by RL. Sahu [15] (36 weeks).

Table 19: Consolidation of humeral shaft fractures treated by centromedullary nailing.

Author	Number of cases	Consolidation (%)	Consolidation time (weeks)
RL. Sahu [15]	78/78	77/78	36
M.J.G Blyth [23]	50/50	43/50	16,8
K. Singisetti [19]	20/36	10/20	16

V.2.2.2. Complications :

V.2.2.2.1. Sepsis :

In the literature the frequency of sepsis after treatment is 1.15% [15, 19, 21-23, 25].

V.2.2.2.2. Pseudarthrosis :

In the literature, the incidence of pseudarthrosis after treatment with centromedullary nailing is 5.34% [15, 19, 21-23, 25] .

V.2.2.2.3. Secondary radial paralysis :

In the literature, the frequency of secondary radial paralysis after treatment with centromedullary nailing was 4.68% [15, 19, 21- 23, 25].Delayed consolidation: In the literature, the incidence of delayed consolidation after treatment with centromedullary nailing was 8.05% [15, 19, 21-...]. 23, 25] .

V.2.2.2.5Vicious cycle :

No fracture consolidated into a vicious callus after treatment with centromedullary nailing [15, 19, 21-23, 25].

Table 20: Complications of diaphyseal fractures treated by centromedullary nailing.

Author	No. of cases	Pseudarthrosis	Radial paralysis	Sepsis	Delayed consolidation	Vicious callus
RL. Sahu [15]	78/78	4/78	0	0	5/78	0
B. D'Ythurbide [21]	57/57	4/57	1/57	1/57	0	0
M.J.G Blyth [23]	51/51	3/51	8/51	0	0	0
K. Singisetti[19]	20/36	1/20	0	1/20	10/20	0
AB. Putti [22]	16/34	0	2/16	0	0	0
M.B Gottschalk [25]	870/3480	11/870	27/870	13/870	0	0

V.2.4. Percutaneous pinning :

V.2.3.1. Consolidation :

In the literature, the rate of consolidation in fractures operated on by percutaneous pinning was 76.95% [11-13, 16, 26].

Table 21: Consolidation of humeral shaft fractures treated by percutaneous pinning.

Author	Number of cases	Consolidation	Deadline of consolidation (Weeks)
M.Barsaoui[11]	70/70	60/70	11
O. Margad [13]	70/70	68/70	10
O.Mohamed[12]	51/51	47/51	10
C.B Diémé [16]	58/58	55/58	10
C. Leblanc [26]	53/120	48/53	11

V.2.3.2. Complications :

V.2.3.2.1. Sepsis :

In the literature the frequency of sepsis after treatment was 2.93% [12, 13,16].

V.2.3.2.2. Pseudarthrosis :

In the literature, the incidence of pseudarthrosis after treatment with percutaneous pinning was 11.08% [12, 13, 16]. These were fractures in the lower third of the humeral shaft, one type B1 and the other type A2. Pseudarthroses were treated with screw plates.

V.2.3.2.3. Secondary radial paralysis :

According to C.B. Diémé [16], 5/58 of the cases treated by pinning were complicated by secondary radial paralysis.

V.2.3.2.4. Delayed consolidation :

In the literature, the incidence of delayed consolidation after treatment with percutaneous pinning is 6.55% [12, 13, 16].

V.2.3.2.5. Cal vicious :

In the literature, the incidence of callus after treatment with percutaneous pinning was 28.28% [12, 13, 16], and is well tolerated.

Table22 : Complications in humeral shaft fractures treated by percutaneous pinning.

Author	Nbof Case	Pseud arthrosis	Radial paralysis	Sepsis	Delayed consolidation	Vicious callus
O.Margad[13]	70/70	2/70	0	0	4/70	0
O. Mohamed [12]	51/51	4/51	0	3/51	3/51	0
C.B.Diémé[16]	58/58	3/58	5/58	3/51	4/58	24/58

VI. FUNCTIONAL RESULTS

VI.1. Overall results :

According to Stewart and Hundley's modified classification, bad cases were pseudarthrosis and cases complicated by stiffness of the shoulder and elbow. These results were found in the series by Margad [13] and Sahu [15].

Table 23: Overall results according to Stewart & Hundley

Author	Very good and Coupons	Quite Good	Bad	Number of case
Margad[13]	55	10	5	70
Sahu[15]	66	8	4	78

VI.2.1. Screw-on plate :

Table 24: Overall functional results of fractures treated with target plates

Author	Very good	Good	Fairly good	Bad
K. Singisetti [19]	4/16	11/16	0	1/16

VI.2.2. Centromedullary nailing :

Table 25: Overall functional results of fractures treated by centromedullary nailing

Author	Very good	Good	Fairly good	Bad
RL.Sahu[15]	69/78	5/78		
K. Singisetti[19]	4/20	9/20	5/20	2/20
B. D'Ythurbide[21]	25/57	20/57	5/57	7/57

VI.2.3. Fasciculated pinning :

Table 26: Overall functional results of fractures treated with fasciculated pinning

Author	Very good	Good	Fairly good	Bad
O. Mohamed[12]	42/54	4/54	1/54	4/54
O.Margad[13]	60/80	6/80	2/80	2/80
C.BDiémé[16]	23/58	26/58	5/58	4/58

VI.2. The Quick Dash :

Table 27: Quick Dash score by technique

Author	Plate Screwed	Fasciculated pinning	Centromedullary nailing	Average
N.Nachef [10] (PRND)	1,67 - 82,5	-	-	20,7
N.Nachef [10] (PRD)	30 - 65	-	-	47,8

VI.3. Pain :

33 of the cases in which the fracture had consolidated had no pain at the last recut. 2 cases had permanent pain, both of which were pseudarthroses.

Table 28: Pain at last recoil

Author	Absent	Climate	During exercise	Permanent
B. D' Ythurbide [21]	54	0	0	3

The following decision tree summarises the findings of our study:

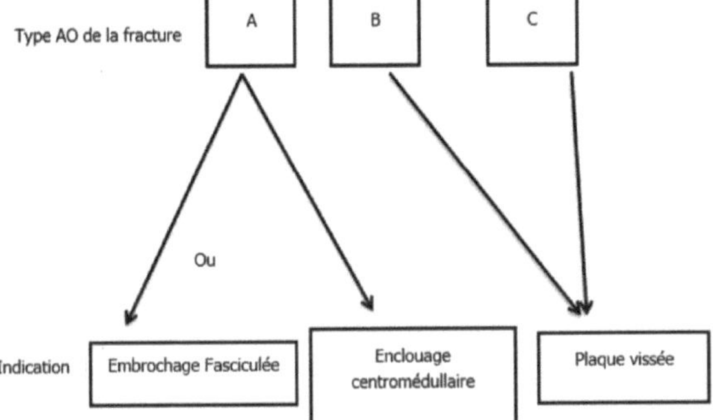

CLINICAL CASE

Clinical case N°1 :

A 33-year-old patient with no prior history was involved in a road traffic accident involving a car skid, resulting in trauma to the left arm with no vascular or nerve complications. The initial radiograph of the left humerus, in front and in profile, showed a type B1 fracture of the lower third of the left humeral shaft.

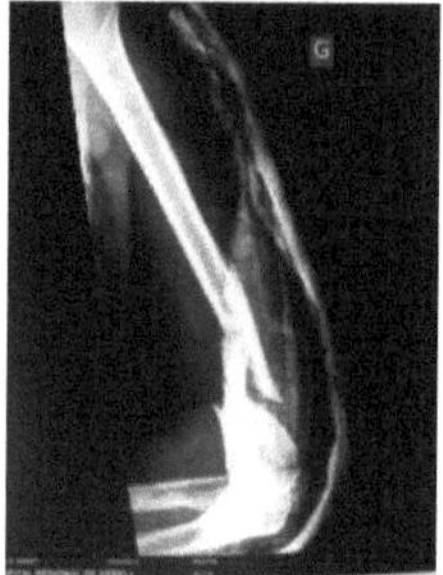

Figure 9: Type B1 fracture of the lower third of the left humeral shaft.

The patient was treated surgically by reduction and osteosynthesis using a screw plate, with a simple post-operative course.

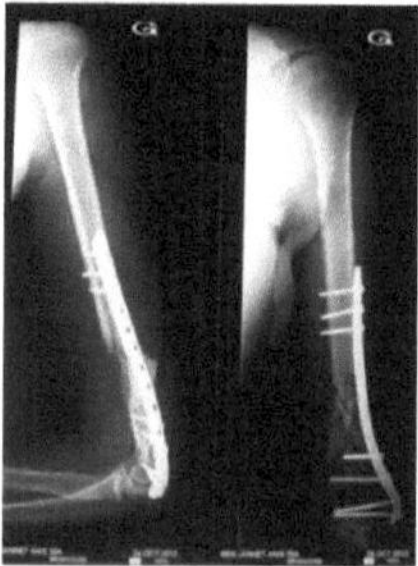

Figure 10: Fracture reduction using a good quality screw plate position.

At the final follow-up of 1 year and 6 months post-operatively, the patient had excellent shoulder and elbow mobility with radiological consolidation. The Quick Dash was 260.

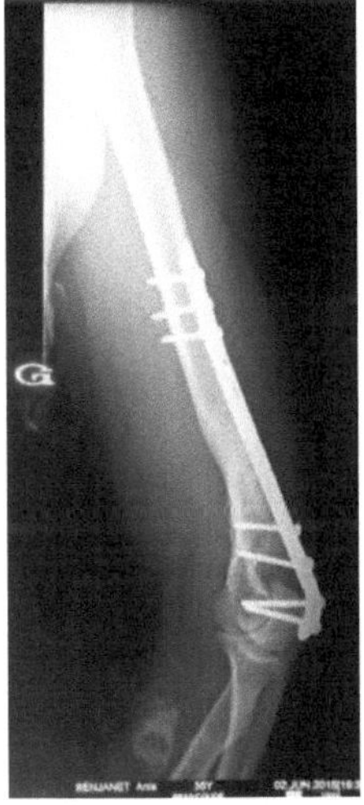

Figure 11: Radiograph of the last recoil.

Clinical case N°2 :

A 39-year-old patient with no previous pathological history was involved in a road traffic accident involving a collision between a car and a lorry, resulting in trauma to the right arm with no vasculo-nervous complications and trauma to the left knee. The initial radiograph of the right humerus from the front and in profile showed a C1 fracture of the mid-diaphysis.

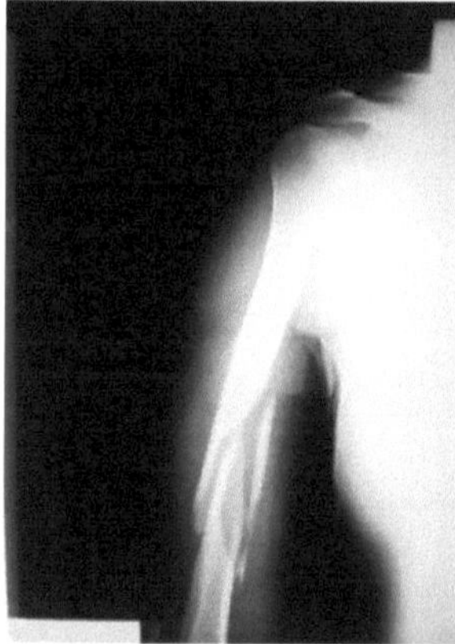

Figure 12: Fracture of the middle third of the humeral shaft C1-type right-hand drive.

The patient underwent reduction surgery and centromedullary nailing for osteosynthesis, with a simple postoperative course.

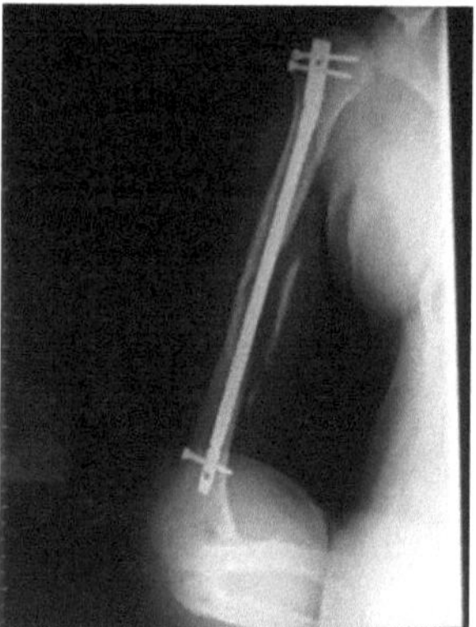

Figure 13: Reduction and osteosynthesis of the fracture by nailing centromedullary.

At the latest follow-up of 4 years, the patient had excellent mobility of the shoulder and elbow, with radiological consolidation. The Quick Dash was 300.

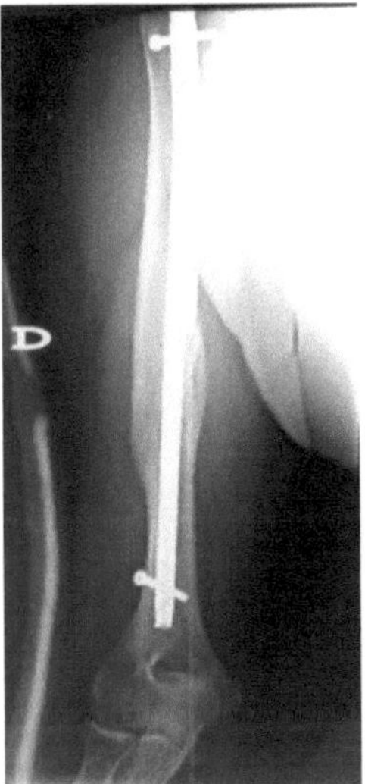

Figure 14: Consolidated fracture in good position.

Clinical case N°3 :

In a 28-year-old patient with no previous history of a road traffic accident, a front-seat passenger in a car collided with another car, resulting in closed trauma to the right upper limb with no vascular or nerve complications. Initial radiographs of the right humerus from the front and in profile showed a fracture of the junction between the middle and lower thirds of the right humerus, with a type B1 3rd fragment.

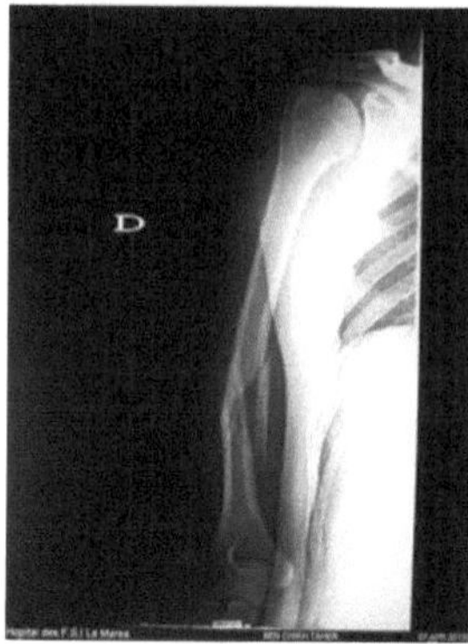

Figure 15: Fracture of the middle-lower third junction of the right humerus type B1.

The patient underwent reduction surgery and fasciculated pinning osteosynthesis with a simple post-operative course.

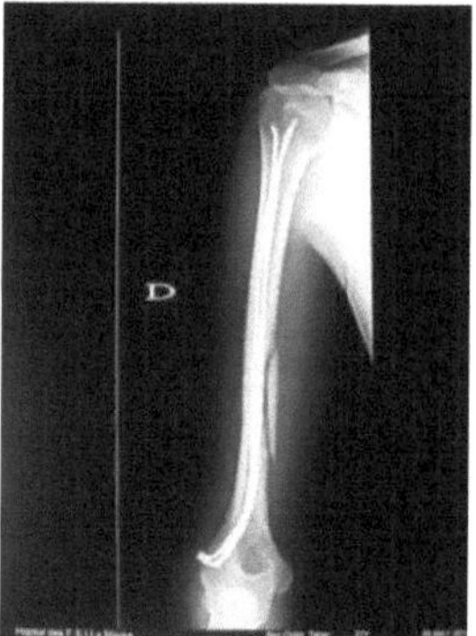

Figure 16: Reduction of the fracture into the correct position by percutaneous pinning.

The last follow-up at 9 months post-operatively showed that the fracture had not yet consolidated.

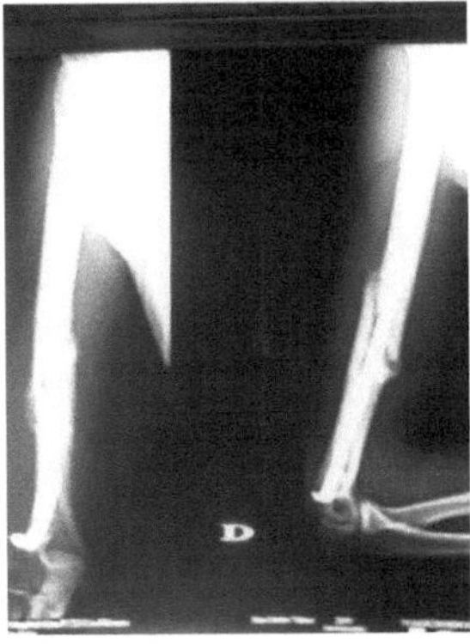

Figure 17: Non-consolidating radiograph.

The patient was operated on again, and his pseudarthrosis was cured with cancellous bone and a screw-retained plate, with a simple post-operative course.

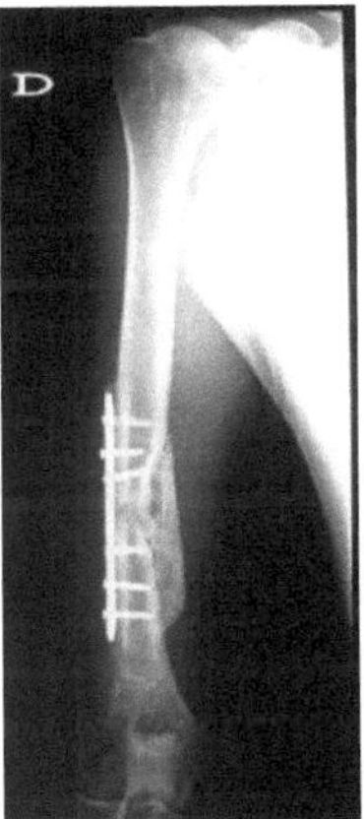

Figure 18: Fracture reduction using a screw plate in good condition position.

At the last follow-up at 3 years, the patient had excellent mobility in the shoulder and elbow, with radiological consolidation. The Quick Dash was 300.

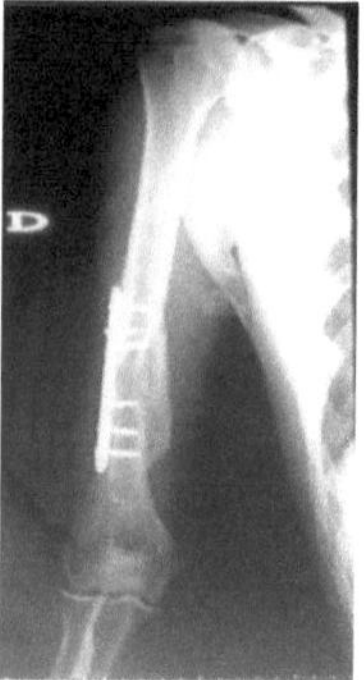

Figure 19: Radiograph of the last recoil.

Clinical case N°4 :

In a 25-year-old patient with no particular history who was involved in a road traffic accident, the front passenger of a car hit a lamppost, resulting in trauma to the right arm complicated by radial paresis. Initial radiographs of the right humerus from the front and in profile revealed an A2 fracture of the lower third of the right humeral shaft.

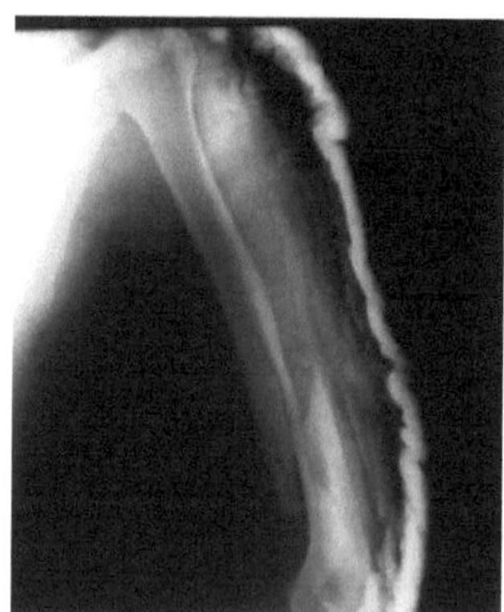

Figure 20: Type A2 fracture of the lower third of the right humeral shaft.

The patient underwent reduction surgery and screw plate osteosynthesis, with intraoperative identification of a contused radial nerve and post-operative clinical observation of radial paralysis. The radial damage was confirmed by an electromyogram and the patient was fitted with a splint on discharge. The radial paralysis recovered after 8 months.

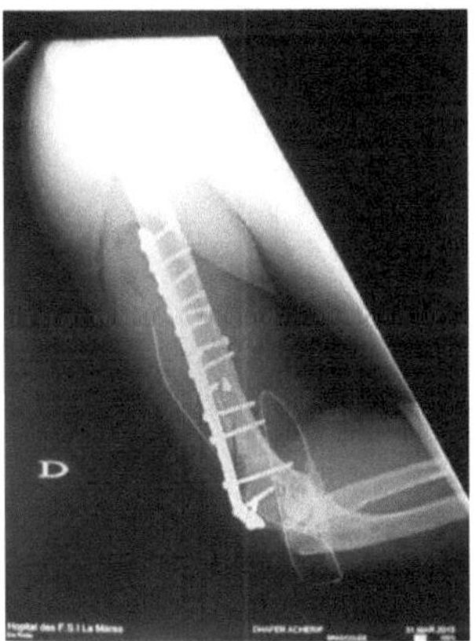

Figure 21: Reduction and osteosynthesis of the fracture using a screw plate.

At the last follow-up of 2 years, the patient was bothered by a protruding screw, no longer had any sensory-motor deficit and had excellent mobility of the shoulder and elbow with radiological consolidation. Quick dash was 300.

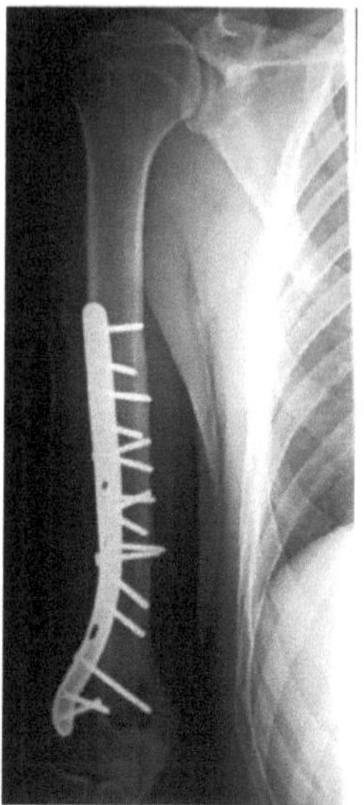

Figure 22: Radiograph of the last recoil.

CONCLUSIONS

In our review of the literature, we assessed the functional results, according to the modified Stewart and Hundley classification, the clinical results, by studying shoulder and elbow mobility, and the radiological results of each type of humeral shaft fracture surgery: fasciculated pinning, screw plate and centromedullary nailing. We found a clear male predominance, and that public road accidents were the main cause of trauma.The fractures were essentially of direct mechanism, their preferred site was the lower third, and their line was most often of type A according to the AO.The overall functional result was good or very good in 85% of cases.Mastery of a technique used routinely by a trained team significantly reduces the risk of complications inherent in each method. The fasciculated pinning technique has numerous indications, particularly in patients with poly fractures or polytrauma, and is applicable to transverse, short oblique, flexion wedge or even bifocal fractures. In addition to the difficulty of reduction and osteosynthesis, the major disadvantages of this technique are that primary stability i s far from optimal and, as a result, additional immobilisation of at least 45 days is required, delaying functional recovery and resumption of work. A rate of Pseudoarthrosis and vicious callus are more frequent than with other techniques, and are associated with the medium-term effects of this technique. Locked centromedullary nailing, an elegant and revolutionary method of osteosynthesis for diaphyseal fractures of the humerus, which, subject to stringent technical requirements and rigour, offers good impaction of the fracture site and excellent primary stability even for the most complex fractures, without touching the fracture site, allowing almost immediate mobilisation, rapid functional recovery with early resumption of work and a better chance of consolidation.Although screw-plate osteosynthesis makes it possible to visualise and control the radial nerve, there is a risk of adverse consequences, often paresis, which recovers in the vast majority of cases within six months of surgery, in addition to the risk of infection. Rigid plate osteosynthesis of diaphyseal fractures of the humerus allows anatomical reduction, good impaction and confrontation of the fragments with excellent primary stability. Open-focus osteosynthesis can be used in monofractured patients, and more often in patients with radial paralysis concomitant with the trauma, but also in patients with stepped trauma of the upper limb, to stabilise transverse, short oblique or distal fractures. Good primary stability is often achieved without the need for light complementary support in the form of a sling for the duration of the injury.2 to 3, resulting in functional recovery and work integration times that are shorter than those for pinning and longer than those for nailing. The persistence of an initial radial paralysis should also prompt a response by requesting an electromyographic check from the 45th day. After six months with no signs of recovery, surgical repair should be considered as soon as the bone has consolidated, with neurolysis of the radial more or less combined with a nerve graft.The humerus may be a forgiving bone, as we said at the beginning of this paper, but when initial treatment fails, it can become difficult to consolidate, requiring both retrospective and prospective reflection in the search for the most appropriate therapeutic solutions.Once again, this highlights the importance of finality and the rigour required to execute the final gesture.Our therapeutic approach depends on the AO type of humeral shaft fracture; for type B or C fractures, we opt for the screw plate. For type A fractures, the treatment is either fasciculated pinning or centromedullary nailing. In order to be able to draw more concrete conclusions, a larger number of people is required, encouraging us to continue our quest for the truth.

REFERENCES

[1] Coudane H, Bonnevialle P, Bernard JN, et al. Fractures de la diaphyse humérale chez l'adulte: EMC Appareil locomoteur.

[2] Barsotti J, Cancel J, Robert C. Guide pratique de traumatologie. (DEPRECIATED), 2010.

[3] Ward EF, Savoie FH, Hughes JL. Fractures of the Diaphyseal Humerus. Skeletal Trauma: Fractures, Dislocation, Ligamentous Injuries.

[4] Borgi R, Butel J, Seringe R, et al. Manuel du traitement orthopédique des fractures des membres et des ceintureurs. Masson, 1981.

[5] Muller B. Étude comparative de l'enclouage de Ender verrouillé et de la vis plaque DHS dans les fractures trochantériennes. PhD Thesis, Thèse médecine, Strasbourg, 1990.

[6] Bonnevialle P. Surgery of the humeral diaphysis: approaches, surgical techniques. Encycl Med Chir.

[7] Seidel H. Traitement des fractures de l'humérus à l'aide du clou verrouillé. Paris: Cahiers d'Enseignement de la SOFCOT Exp Scie Fra 1990; 39: 55-9.

[8] Kempf I, Grosse A, Taglang G, et al. The gamma nail in the closed treatment of trochanteric fractures. Results and indications from a series of 121 cases. Revue de chirurgie orthopédique et traumatologique 2014; 100: 70-79.

[9] Riemer BL, D'Ambrosia R. The risk of injury to the axillary nerve, artery, and vein from proximal locking screws of humeral intramedullary nails. Orthopedics 1992; 15: 697-699.

[10] Nachef N, Bariatinsky V, Sulimovic S, et al. Prognostic factors for recovery of radial palsies in humeral diaphyseal fractures: about 17 cases. Revue de Chirurgie Orthopédique et Traumatologique 2017; 103: 123-128.

[11] Barsaoui M, Msakni A, Zitouna K, et al. Results of treatment of diaphyseal fractures of the humerus by centromedullary embrochage. A review of 70 cases. Revue de Chirurgie Orthopédique et Traumatologique 2014; 100: S249-S250.

[12] Mohamed O, Bousbaa H, Bennani M, et al. Treatment of humeral shaft fractures with Hackethal retrograde centromedullary embrochage: 54 cases. Pan African Medical Journal; 30.

[13] Margad O, Boukhris J, Sallahi H, et al. Place of Hackethal fasciculated pinning in the treatment of humerus fractures: a review of 80 cases. The Pan African Medical Journal; 24.

[14] Ring D, Chin K, Jupiter JB. Radial nerve palsy associated with high-energy humeral shaft fractures. The Journal of hand surgery 2004; 29: 144-147.

[15] Sahu RL, Ranjan R, Lal A. Fracture union in closed interlocking nail in humeral shaft fractures. Chinese Medical Journal 2015; 128: 1428-1432.

[16] Diémé CB, Abalo A, Sané AD, et al. Ascending centromedullary embrochage of diaphyseal fractures of the adult humerus. Evaluation of anatomical and functional results in 63 cases. Chirurgie de la main 2005; 24: 92-98.

[17] Flinkkilä T, Hyvönen P, Lakovaara M, et al. Intramedullary nailing of humeral shaft fractures: a retrospective study of 126 cases. Acta orthopaedica Scandinavica 1999; 70: 133-136.

[18] Bèzes H. The value of screw-plate fixation of many humeral shaft fractures: a review of 246 cases. International orthopaedics 1995; 19: 16-25.

[19] Singisetti K, Ambedkar M. Nailing versus plating in humerus shaft fractures: a prospective comparative study. International orthopaedics 2010; 34: 571-576.

[20] Foster RJ, Swiontkowski MF, Bach AW, et al. Radial nerve palsy caused by open humeral shaft fractures. The Journal of hand surgery 1993; 18: 121-124.

[21] D'YTHURBIDE B, Augereau B, Asselineau A, et al. High approach centromedullary locking of recent humeral shaft fractures. International orthopaedics 1983; 7: 195-203.

[22] Putti AB, Uppin RB, Putti BB. Locked intramedullary nailing versus dynamic compression plating for humeral shaft fractures. Journal of Orthopaedic Surgery 2009; 17: 139-141.

[23] Blyth MJG, Macleod CMB, Asante DK, et al. Iatrogenic nerve injury with the Russell-Taylor humeral nail. Injury 2003; 34: 227-228.

[24] Chapman JR, Henley MB, Agel J, et al. Randomized prospective study of humeral shaft fracture fixation: intramedullary nails versus plates. Journal of orthopaedic trauma 2000; 14: 162-166.

[25] Gottschalk MB, Carpenter W, Hiza E, et al. Humeral shaft fracture fixation: incidence rates and complications as reported by American Board of Orthopaedic Surgery part II candidates. JBJS 2016; 98: e71.

[26] Clowez G, Gastaud O, Djian M, et al. Centromedullary nailing for humeral shaft fracture, is distal locking essential? Revue de Chirurgie Orthopédique et Traumatologique 2016; 102: S149.

TABLE OF CONTENTS

FRACTURES OF THE HUMERAL SHAFT 1

I.EPIDEMIOLOGY 9

II.PREOPERATIVE RESULTS 11

III.TREATMENT 15

IV.POSTOPERATIVE RESULTS 18

V.RESULTS AT LAST RETREAT 19

VI.FUNCTIONAL RESULTS.....................................26

CLINICAL CASE 30

CONCLUSIONS...39

REFERENCES...41

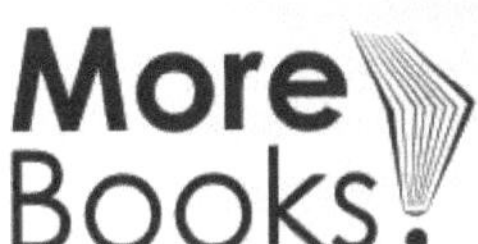

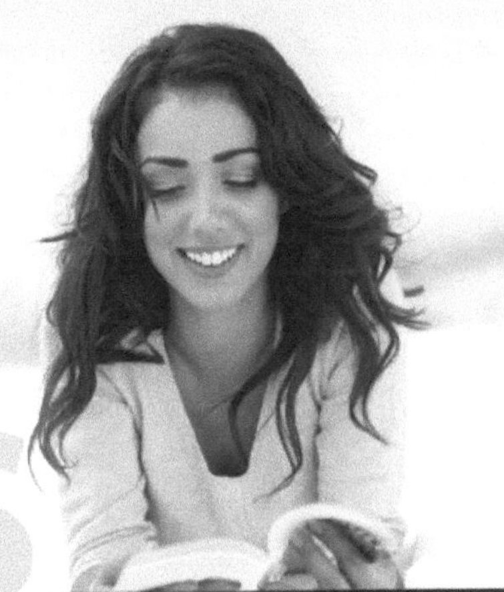

yes
I want morebooks!

Buy your books fast and straightforward online - at one of world's fastest growing online book stores! Environmentally sound due to Print-on-Demand technologies.

Buy your books online at
www.morebooks.shop

Kaufen Sie Ihre Bücher schnell und unkompliziert online – auf einer der am schnellsten wachsenden Buchhandelsplattformen weltweit! Dank Print-On-Demand umwelt- und ressourcenschonend produziert.

Bücher schneller online kaufen
www.morebooks.shop

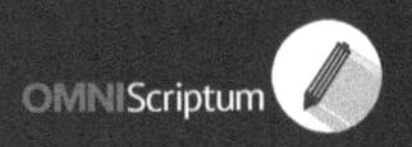

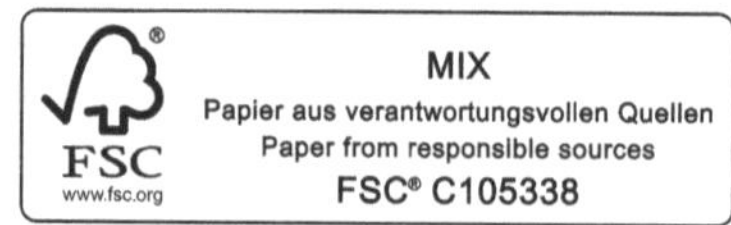

Printed by Books on Demand GmbH, Norderstedt / Germany